LEARN HOW TO USE (ASPIRIN)

Understanding its Role in Cardiovascular Health, Cancer Prevention and More

Dr. Kamil Dragutin

Table of Contents

CHAPTER ONE

Introduction to Aspirin

Of all medications taken and studied, aspirin is formally known as acetylsalicylic acid, ASA, and is probably one of the most consumed and well-researched. It forms a group called nonsteroidal anti-inflammatory drugs, NSAIDs. Mostly, it is prescribed because of its analgesic, antipyretic, and anti-inflammatory effects. The primary role of this medicine is in the prevention and treatment of cardiovascular diseases through its antiplatelet effects.

History and Development

Aspirin has its history as far back as ancient times when willow bark and leaves, containing salicin, were used for analgesia and to bring down fever. In 1828, the German chemist Johann Buchner was able to isolate salicin in its pure form. By 1897, Bayer chemist Felix Hoffmann had synthesized acetylsalicylic acid in a stable form, more handleable as a drug. Bayer launched it as "Aspirin," and it took rapid acceptance worldwide.

Chemical Composition and Properties

The chemical formula for aspirin is $C_9H_8O_4$, with a molecular weight of 180.16

g/mol. It is a white, fine, crystalline powder with a slightly bitter taste. Aspirin is relatively stable in its solid form but hydrolyzes into salicylic acid and acetic acid in the presence of moisture. This hydrolysis can be minimized by proper storage in dry conditions.

Mechanism of Action

The main action of aspirin is via the inhibition of the enzyme cyclooxygenase

(COX). This enzyme has two main isoforms: COX-1 and COX-2. Aspirin irreversibly inhibits COX-1 and COX-2, thus blocking the formation of prostaglandins and thromboxanes from arachidonic acid.

Prostaglandins mediate inflammation, pain, and fever.

Thromboxane A2 has an established role in platelet aggregation and vasoconstriction.

If inhibited, these pathways give aspirin its anti-inflammatory, analgesic, antipyretic, and antiplatelet properties.

Medical Applications of Aspirin

Aspirin is remarkably effective against mild to moderate pain, such as headache, toothache, muscle pain, and arthritis. It reduces pain by blocking the production of prostaglandins, which sensitize pain receptors.

Anti-inflammatory Effects

Aspirin is applied in conditions like rheumatoid arthritis, osteoarthritis, and other inflammatory disorders because it has anti-inflammatory properties. It decreases inflammation, swelling, and soreness in the joints.

Cardiovascular Benefits

The most useful applications of aspirin are in the prevention and treatment of cardiovascular diseases. The low dose of aspirin (usually 75-100 mg) prevents blood clotting and reduces the risk of heart attack or stroke. It is indicated in:

Patients who have already had a myocardial infarction or stroke. These are potential candidates for secondary prevention with aspirin.

Patients at high risk for experiencing a

cardiovascular event. This indication is more controversial and should be weighed on an individual basis.

Other Uses

Aspirin has been evaluated for many other medical

disorders. This includes the following:

Colorectal Cancer Prevention

Several studies have reported that long-term use of low-dose aspirin might reduce the risk of

Low dose as aspirin is sometimes indicated in

pregnant women at high risk of developing preeclampsia for its prevention.

CHAPTER TWO

Dosage and Administration

The dose of aspirin would depend on the condition to be treated:

In the case of pain and fever, 325-650 mg every 4-

6 hours as required; not to exceed 4 grams per day

The usual dose is higher, 2-3 grams per day in divided doses

Low dose aspirin, usually 75-100 mg once daily to prevent cardiovascular issues.

The aspirin should be taken with food or a full glass of water to minimize gastrointestinal discomfort. There is also enteric-coated aspirin, which can be taken to lower gastric irritation.

Side Effects and Adverse Reactions

Although aspirin is safe when taken as recommended, it frequently causes adverse side effects, especially when taken in large quantities or over a long period. It often causes the following side effects, including:

Gastrointestinal effects: Nausea, vomiting, stomach pain, heartburn.

Aspirin exhibits an antiplatelet effect, which increases the risk of bleeding, including gastrointestinal bleeding and bruising.

Hives, rash, swelling, and rarely, anaphylaxis

Ringing in the ears; this is more common at higher doses

More serious adverse reactions, though uncommon, can include:

Reye's Syndrome; which is a very rare but serious condition occurring in children and teenagers recovering from viral infections. It is characterized by swelling in the liver and brain.

Stomach or intestinal ulcers are caused by its use for a very long time. Kidney function might get affected due to large doses.

Interactions with Other Medications

Aspirin is a drug interacting with several classes of medication, either altering their actions or increasing the risk of side effects. These include:

- **Anticoagulant medications (e.g., Warfarin):** Increased risk for bleeding.

- **Nonsteroidal Anti-Inflammatory Drugs (NSAIDs):** Gastrointestinal bleeding and the reduced effectiveness of both drugs. The risk of gastrointestinal ulcers and bleeding is increased.

Aspirin can reduce the efficiency of some antihypertensive medications.

The toxicity of methotrexate is enhanced because of decreased clearance.

Contraindications and Precautions

Aspirin is contraindicated in some conditions and requires precautions in others. In patients with a history of hypersensitivity to aspirin or other NSAIDs, it is contraindicated. The risk of gastrointestinal bleeding is increased.

There could be increased risk of bleeding. Some asthmatics may experience bronchospasm with aspirin Renal or Hepatic Impairment requires dose adjustment and careful monitoring.

Generally avoided, especially in the third trimester due to potential risks to the fetus

Aspirin is generally not recommended for kids and adolescents, as it could result in Reye's syndrome, a very rare but serious disease.

In general, aspirin is avoided during pregnancy, particularly during the third trimester of pregnancy, due to risks to the fetus and problems at birth. Low-dose aspirin may be given in some high-risk pregnancy cases under medical supervision.

Aspirin is distributed in small amounts in breast milk, and nursing patients should consult a physician. Elderly patients have an increased risk of adverse reactions; specifically, gastrointestinal bleeding and renal impairment. Lower doses and cautious monitoring   are

recommended.

Alternatives to Aspirin

Analgesia   and

antiinflammatory   effect

with reduced doses, less GI bleeding.

Naproxen; which is long-acting; analgesic and antiinflammatory action.

Paracetamol (Acetaminophen) is quite effective against pain and fever, but causes less GI adverse effects. However, it does not have anti-inflammatory action; furthermore, it can cause hepatic toxicity when ingested in large amounts. Clopidogrel is a good alternative to aspirin in patients with intolerance to aspirin or those having recurrent exacerbation of gastrointestinal bleeding to prevent blood clotting.

THE END